Carbs

The No-Bullshit Guide to Ultimate Fat-Loss Transformation through the Use of Strategic Carbohydrate Timing and Techniques

By <Sam Hill >

Disclaimer Notice:

Please note the information contained within this document is for educational purposes only.

Every attempt has been made to provide accurate, up to date and reliable complete information no warranties of any kind are expressed or implied. Readers acknowledge that the author is not engaging in rendering legal, financial or professional advice.

By reading any document, the reader agrees that under no circumstances are we responsible for any losses, direct or indirect, which are incurred as a result of use of the information contained within this document, including – but not limited to errors, omissions, or inaccuracies.

Table of Contents

Introduction

Have you been struggling to lose weight? Are you doing all the right things and still not seeing the results you want? Is your body just not responding to your efforts?

If that's the case, you're not alone. In fact, these frustrations are very common among people who want to lose weight – and that's no surprise. Confusion and irritation occur because there is so much conflicting advice out there. One popular diet tells you that eliminating carbs is the answer, while another does its best to turn dietary fat into the enemy. Still another might tell you to eliminate dairy, or gluten, or to turn to a liquid diet to get rid of those extra pounds.

What do all of these plans have in common? They are all bullshit. Most diet plans are invented by scam artists who are interested in only one thing: earning money. They want to convince you to buy their books, eat their tasteless pre-packaged food, or buy their supplements because they know that you're vulnerable. You want to lose weight, and you're frustrated and disheartened. In other words, you're a good target.

The good news is that there is another way. Food isn't your enemy – and that includes carbs and fats. The goal of this eBook is to give you the information you need to lose weight in a common sense way that's backed by scientific research.

What You Will Learn in This Book

By the time you're done reading this book, you will have all the information you need to lose weight the smart way. We'll cover:

- Why the first thing you need to address is your mindset
- How macronutrients (carbs, proteins and fats) work in your body
- How to tell the difference between good carbs and bad carbs
- How to tell the difference between healthy fats and unhealthy fats
- Why you can't lose weight in the long run without exercise
- Why the timing of what you eat (especially carbs) matters
- How to make a few delicious, low-carb meals that will satisfy you

In addition to all of the above, you'll also get a detailed, 14-day plan to get you started on the road to weight loss. Depending on the amount of weight you need to lose, you may need longer – but 14 days is long enough to detoxify your body and get you accustomed to your new routine.

What you will read in the coming pages is a common sense, scientifically-backed, no-bullshit plan to help you finally lose the weight you want to lose. I hope you're ready, because this plan is about to change your life.

Let's get started.

<u>Chapter 1 – Mind over Matter</u>

What's in your mind when you think about losing weight? If your head is not in the right place, it's going to be very difficult for you to make the changes you need to make to lose weight. In this chapter, we will talk about why that is – and what you can do to achieve the proper mindset for weight loss.

Why Your Brain Must Be on Board if You Want to Change Your Body

No doubt you have heard the expression, "It's a question of mind over matter." People say it so often that it's become a cliché – but a saying only becomes a cliché if it contains something true. The reason your mindset matters it that every single thing that happens in your body is managed by your brain. Now,

11 |

I'm not suggesting that if you tell yourself you will lose weight you can do it without making any changes. However, I am saying that you can't expect to make (and stick to) those changes if you don't have the proper attitude.

One of the biggest mistakes people make when starting a diet plan is that they tell themselves some variation of this: *I only have to do this for a short amount of time and then I can go back to eating whatever I want*. Does that sound familiar? I'm betting it does, and saying things like that to yourself is a sure-fire way to guarantee that you'll fail.

Your body is a complex system, and the things you eat make a big difference in how it looks and works. If eating a certain way has led to you gaining weight, believing that you can go back to that way of life after you lose weight is a recipe for disaster. You have to make a strong decision that you are going to change the way you eat and give your body the fuel it needs to shed fat and look great. That's a decision that has to inform the rest of your life, not just the few weeks or months it takes for you to shed unwanted pounds.

Tips for Achieving the Right Mindset

Getting your head on straight regarding weight loss can be hard, but here are some pointers that may help:

- Stop using the word "diet" and embrace the idea that you are learning about the best fuel to give your body. You wouldn't give your car diesel fuel if it needed unleaded, or go through periods where you gave it the wrong fuel. Give your body the same respect.
- Make a commitment to pay attention to the way your body feels. Many of us ignore the signals our bodies send us, but if we listen those signals can help us figure out the foods that are best for us.
- Don't think of food as the enemy. It's not. You need food to survive. You need

carbohydrates, fats, and proteins to be healthy. Without them, your body cannot function properly.

- Accept that you are human and may occasionally slip – and learn to look at those slips as mistakes, not failures. You can have a slice of birthday cake, just don't let it derail your weight loss efforts.

If you can get the above thoughts into your mind and really believe them, you are well on your way to having the proper mindset to help you lose weight.

Now that you've got your head on straight, let's talk about the basic building blocks of nutrition: macronutrients.

Chapter 2 – Macronutrients and Your Body

The foods you eat are comprised of three major types known as macronutrients. The prefix macro- tells us that these form the majority of your diet. The other key nutritional components of your diet are micronutrients, more commonly known as vitamins and minerals. Your body requires very small amounts of these substances, and healthy macronutrients contain them in sufficient quantities.

What Are Macronutrients?

The three types of macronutrients are carbohydrates, proteins, and fats. Let's talk briefly about each one.

Carbs

Carbohydrates are sugars. It is important to note that not all sugars are bad. We will talk more later about the way that consuming carbohydrates affects your body, but for now what you need to know is that carbohydrates are your body's first source of energy. What that means is that, when you eat carbohydrates, your body will burn them before it accesses other forms of energy. It is for this reason that long-distance runners do a certain amount of carb-loading before a race. It's a way of providing their bodies with extra fuel.

Some dietary sources of carbohydrates include fruits, vegetables, whole grains, starches, table sugar, flour, honey, maple syrup, agave, and other natural sweeteners. *Proteins* are the building blocks of muscle and bone. They are composed of amino acids, with different foods containing different combinations of amino acids. Certain foods, such as quinoa and whole wheat bread with peanut butter, contain all 20 amino acids and are thus referred to as "complete proteins."

Proteins are fibrous and take longer to digest than carbohydrates. Eating proteins keeps you feeling full, making it easy to resist the temptation of snacking between meals. Meat, poultry, and fish are all good sources of protein, as are eggs and milk. Vegetarian protein sources include beans and legumes. Soy beans are an especially popular source of vegetable protein and are the primary ingredient in meat substitutes like tofu.

Fats are also known as lipids. Like proteins, they tend to keep the body satiated and reduce hunger. Eating fats releases a hormone called leptin, which is also known as the satiety hormone.

Like carbohydrates, there are several kinds of fat. Monounsaturated fats are vegetable fats and healthy for your body. Polyunsaturated fats also come from vegetables. Saturated fats come from meats and other animal products. By far the least healthy kind of fat is something called trans fat. If you look at a food label and see ingredients like partially hydrogenated oil, that is a trans fat. Trans fats have been linked to heart disease.

Your body needs all three kinds of macronutrients in the proper ratios to be healthy.

<u>Chapter 3 – Not All Carbs Are Enemies</u>

Now that you understand the basic building blocks of nutrition, it's time to dig a bit deeper into the subject of carbohydrates. Which carbohydrates are good, which are bad, and what do they do to your body when you eat them?

Good Carbs versus Bad Carbs

The first thing you need to know about carbohydrates is that they are not bad for you. It's easy to understand why you might think they are, what with the huge number of products that claim to be low-carb. Remember what I said in the previous chapter: carbohydrates are your body's first source of energy. Your brain needs carbohydrates to function – it's just that simple.

The reason that carbohydrates have got a bad reputation is that we are in love with sugar. A quick perusal of any food label will show you that most processed foods contain an appalling amount of added sugar. It hides under dozens of different names. For example, anything ending with the suffixes – ose or –itol is a sugar. Examples include high fructose corn syrup, maltose, maltitol, and sorbitol.

Refined and simple sugars are what most nutritionists would agree are bad carbs. They offer little in the way of nutritional value and they have a disproportionately high impact on your blood sugar. Naturally-occurring carbs, such as those found in vegetables and fruits, come with a healthy dose of fiber and other nutrients, and they have a minimal effect on your blood sugar. There are the kinds of carbohydrates your body needs to function.

Understanding the Glycemic Index

One of the ways you can measure the healthiness of a carbohydrate is by looking at its glycemic index. The glycemic index is a way of measuring the effect a food has on your blood sugar on a scale from 1 to 100. It was developed by Dr. David J. Jenkins and his colleagues at the University of Toronto in the early 1980s as part of an effort to determine the best diet for people with diabetes. The lower the glycemic index is, the smaller the effect it has on your blood sugar. For example, foods with a high GI tend to cause a rapid spike in blood sugar. The presence of sugar in your blood triggers the release of insulin, an important hormone. Foods with a low GI take longer to digest and release sugar into the bloodstream at a slow and steady rate.

When a person consumes too many foods with a high GI, it can lead to insulin resistance, a condition that can ultimately cause diabetes.

How Eating the Right Carbohydrates Affects Your Body

You know now that eating foods with a high GI causes your blood glucose to increase quickly. It triggers the release of insulin, and if you eat enough sugar, your body can become resistant to the effects of insulin. But what happens when you eat healthy carbohydrates?

When you eat healthy carbohydrates, those with a low glycemic index, the sugars in them are released into your bloodstream slowly. Instead of providing you with a huge boost on energy and blood sugar all at once, they provide you with a slow and steady supply of sugar to your bloodstream. That means that you don't get a big spike of insulin, which keeps your blood sugar steady and you supplied with the energy you need.

Later in the book, I will tell you about the specific timing of when to eat carbohydrates, but next, let's talk about the kinds of fat you need to incorporate into your diet.

Chapter 4 – Fat: Friend or Foe?

Just as carbohydrates have been vilified by the diet industry, the same is true of fats. Fat was actually the enemy before carbs. During the 1990s, supermarket shelves were flooded with low-fat products that people bought over and over again. The problem with that is that the fat was usually replaced with additional sugar (bad carbs) or chemicals (just plain bad.) These foods weren't any healthier than their counterparts, but the food and diet industries did a great job of selling them as if they were.

Good Fats versus Bad Fats

The first thing you need to understand about fats is that they are not all bad. The fats that have a bad reputation are saturated fats, like the kind that comes from meat and animal products, and trans fats, which are processed fats. A trans fat is usually a fat that is liquid at room temperature (think vegetable oil, corn oil, and canola oil) that is processed to turn it into a solid. They are also referred to as partially hydrogenated oils, and examples include margarine and vegetable shortening. According to the American Heart Association, they raise your LDL (bad) cholesterol and decrease your HDL (good) cholesterol. They increase your risk of experiencing a heart attack or stroke. The same is true of saturated fats. The difference is that saturated fat is not avoidable (even some monounsaturated fats like olive oil contain small amounts of saturated fat) while trans fats are. Good fats help keep your digestive system and connective joints lubricated and can decrease your cholesterol.

How Eating the Right Fats Can Help You Lose Weight

The key to including fat in your diet is to eat the proper amount of healthy fat. As I stated above, healthy fats help keep your heart strong, your cholesterol in check, and your body lubricated. They also help you feel satisfied by the food you eat, something that's very important when you're cutting calories.

A 2015 article in Scientific American talked about why fat is so important to health. Eating monounsaturated and polyunsaturated fats, and keeping your total intake to about 30% of your daily calories, helps promote good heart and joint health. It is also extremely important for proper brain function. 60% of your brain tissue is composed of fat, so eating a diet that's too low in fat can starve your brain. Considering that your brain controls everything that happens in your body, including hormone production, energy levels, and distribution of nutrients, this is not a small thing. People who eat a diet rich in the proper kinds of fat have a significantly lower risk of dementia than those who eat a low-fat diet.

Eating the right kind of fat actually makes it easy for you to lose weight. The healthy fats you eat trigger the release of leptin, a hormone that makes you feel full and satisfied. That means that you're less likely to overeat or snack between meals. Fat also adds flavor to food which decreases the likelihood that you will feel deprived. And because it improves your heart function, it will make your exercise productive and ensure that you have the energy to complete your workouts on a regular basis.

Chapter 5 – Why Movement Matters

So far, the focus of this book has been on the changes you need to make to your diet in order to lose weight. Many people who want to lose weight would prefer not to have to worry about exercise, but the fact is that you won't be able to lose weight permanently unless you get your body moving.

Why Exercise and Weight Training Are Necessary

The first thing you need to understand about exercise is what it does to your body. People gain weight because they take in more calories than they burn. You must take in 3,500 more calories than you burn to gain one pound of weight. In simple terms, if you eat 500 extra calories a day, you will gain one pound in a week.

The benefit of exercise is that it helps you to burn more calories. It increases your metabolism and makes it easier for you to lose weight. If you want to lose weight, you need to give your body healthy fuel – the right carbohydrates, fats, and proteins – and keep it active. And while it might seem contradictory, exercising gives you extra energy.

The Benefits of Different Kinds of Exercise

Specific types of exercise have different benefits. Let's take a quick look at what some popular workouts can do for your body:

- **Cardio.** When you do cardio work, you elevate your heart rate and improve your circulation. You also burn calories. As we discussed previously, your body will burn available carbohydrates first, and then it will burn fat. The longer you exercise, the more likely you are to burn fat. Examples of cardio exercises include walking, running, biking, and swimming.
- **Strength training.** Strength training (usually with weights) burns some calories too, but its primary function is building up muscle in your body. Not

only will that help you have a shapelier, more toned body, but muscle burns more calories when you are at rest than fat does.

- **Toning.** Workouts like yoga, Pilates, t'ai chi, and others work by toning your muscles, increasing flexibility, and improving the connection between your body and mind. They burn some calories, but not as many as cardio exercise does.

- **Team sports.** Some people prefer to work out alone, while others like the camaraderie of participating in a team sport such as softball, soccer, or even Ultimate Frisbee.

Whatever form of exercise you choose, it is important to do it at least three or four times a week for 30 minutes at a time. The more you exercise, the more calories you will burn and the more weight you will lose.

Chapter 6 – Timing Is Everything

By now you're probably wondering how to put all of the information I've given you about eating carbs and fat together in a coherent way to help you lose weight. When you're stuck, it's easy to get frustrated – especially if you've been cutting way back on calories and exercising too. If you're hungry all the time, then you probably feel like you should be losing weight. In this chapter, I'll tell you about one of the most common reasons why people fail to lose weight even though they're cutting calories.

When to Eat Carbs to Lose Weight

When you're thinking about carbs and weight loss, it is important to know which carbs are healthy and which are not. However, it's not just about the quality of the carbs you eat – the timing matters, too. Here's what I'm talking about:

1. Your body's calorie-burning potential is higher earlier in the day. If you're going to eat starchy carbs such as whole grains, potatoes, or rice, it's best to do it early in the day so you have plenty of time to work them off. The reason this works is that you are active during the day, whether you're working out, or just running errands or doing housework. A recent study from Northwestern

University showed that people who ate later in the day (having their last meal after 8:00 pm) consumed 248 more calories per day than those who got up earlier and ate earlier. 248 calories a day adds up to about one extra pound every two weeks.

2. It is also a good idea to eat carbohydrates after you work out. A 1999 study at Appalachian State University tested athletes' stores of glycogen (the name for stored glucose in the body) before and after a workout, and found that glycogen stores were reduced during exercise. That makes sense because when you work out, especially for an extended period of time, your body burns glycogen to keep going. Eating complex carbohydrates about 45 minutes after you work out can

help your body replenish its stores of glycogen. Because your metabolism is high after you work out, eating carbs at this time decreases the chances that the glucose in what you eat will be stored as fat and increases the chances it will be stored as glycogen.

3. The timing of food in general is important. People who get enough sleep, get up early, and stop eating early in the day are significantly less likely to become obese than people who get inadequate sleep and eat late in the day.

As you can see, the timing of what you eat matters, and that's something that will come into play in the next chapter.

Hormones and Weight Loss

The final thing you need to understand before we move on to discussing the specific 14-day plan to help you lose weight is the role that hormones play in weight loss. There are five main hormones that have to do with diet and metabolism:

1. Insulin. Insulin is the hormone that your body releases when you consume carbohydrates or sugars. Its role is to help distribute the glucose in your blood to the parts of your body that need it. It also plays a role in how your body stores excess glucose as glycogen. People who eat too much sugar can end up with insulin resistance, which can develop into Type II diabetes. Some

people cannot produce insulin at all, and they have Type I diabetes.

2. Ghrelin is a hormone that is released by your digestive system when your stomach is empty and you are hungry. For this reason, it is known as the "hunger hormone." Typically when you eat and your stomach stretches, your body's production of ghrelin stops. Sometimes people produce excess ghrelin, which causes them to eat even when they are not hungry.

3. Glucagon is the hormone that your body releases when you eat protein. Glucagon has the opposite effect to insulin – in other words, it increases the concentration of glucose in the blood. Eating protein and carbs together can help keep blood sugar levels under control.

4. Cholecystokinin is a hormone that your body releases when you eat fat. It suppresses the body's production of ghrelin and reduces your hunger.

5. Leptin is the so-called 'satiety hormone' that lets you know when you have had enough to eat. Sometimes, people who are obese can become resistant to leptin, and that causes them to overeat.

When you are trying to lose weight, it is very important to keep your hormones in balance. That means eating the proper ratios of micronutrients so that your blood sugar is under control and you have a slow-releasing source of energy that keeps you going through the day. That is what we'll talk about in the next chapter.

Chapter 7 – The No-Bullshit Plan to Lose Weight

Now it's time to put everything we've discussed so far together into an easy-to-follow, no-bullshit plan that will help you break out of your rut and lose weight. The focus here will be on how much to eat and when to eat it, and then in the next chapter I'll give you a few easy recipes and some general diet tips to get you started.

The Basics

Before I break down the plan, let's talk about some important basics for weight loss:

1. Get enough sleep. Research shows that insufficient sleep can lead to weight gain. Your brain uses the time you are

sleeping to clear out biochemical waste, and sleeping gives your body a chance to recuperate. Aim for seven or eight hours per night, and try to stick to a regular sleep schedule.

2. Drink enough water. Hydration is very important for weight loss, and most of us don't get enough water. You need to drink at least 64 ounces of water per day, and you may need more if you are very tall, very overweight, or very active. If you live in a warm climate, make sure to drink extra water to compensate for what you lose when you perspire.

3. Remember to keep the proper mindset as discussed earlier in the book. The food you eat is fuel for your body. Of course, you want it to be delicious, but it is important to put deliciousness second to what the food you eat can do to you.

You can make any healthy, natural food tasty if you prepare it properly.

These three things – sleep, hydration, and mindset – must be constants. If you ignore them, you will not be able to lose weight.

The final thing you must do to prepare is to go through the food you currently have in your pantry and kitchen and get rid of the foods that are preventing you from losing weight. For example:

- Foods with added sugar (look for anything ending in –ose or –itol)
- Foods with artificial sweeteners
- Foods with trans fat
- Foods with monosodium glutamate (MSG)

If you are accustomed to eating a diet high in these foods, be aware that your body may experience some withdrawal symptoms. That's normal, and it's part of the reason why it's so important to have the proper mindset. When you feel an intense craving for sugar or anything else unhealthy, try sipping tea or chewing a piece of sugarless gum. You can also eat a healthy, low-carb snack such as celery sticks or radishes.

The Plan

The first thing you need to know, because it will remain consistent throughout the plan, is how to break down your macronutrient consumption. In general, you want to get:

- No more than 25% carb-dense foods (these are foods like grains, starches, and refined sugars). If you have a lot of weight to lose, you should minimize these foods as much as possible.
- 25-30% low glycemic index carbs such as fruits and vegetables
- 25-30% healthy fat
- Between 20% and 40% protein, depending on your intake of carb-dense foods.

Remember that carb-dense foods tend to reduce the amount of protein you need. The best time to eat carb-dense foods is early in the day, and preferably after a workout. Your metabolism is in full gear after a workout, and when it's early in the day you can be confident that you'll have plenty of time to burn the carbs you eat. The amount of time you have after a workout to consume carb-dense foods depends on the intensity of your workout. For a very intense workout such as a marathon or other endurance workout, you should replenish your body's carbs within 30 minutes. For low- or medium-intensity workouts, you have about two or three hours to replenish. That might seem counterintuitive, but long workouts deplete the body's stores of glycogen and the longer you wait to refuel, the longer it will take you to recover properly.

Week One

Start each day with a healthy breakfast, such as a breakfast burrito (recipe in the next chapter) or even something simple like whole wheat toast with natural peanut butter. This combination forms a complete protein and will keep you satisfied for hours.

If possible, get your workout in before lunch. Remember, you want to get at least 30 minutes of aerobic activity three to four times a week. If you have been very sedentary before now, start with something low impact, like walking, and work your way up to something more strenuous. Eat a workout-recovery meal like the quinoa salad in the next chapter as soon as possible after your workout.

Eat a meal of healthy carbohydrates like vegetables, along with lean protein and healthy fat, for dinner. Eat your final meal of the day before 8:00 (earlier if possible) and try drinking tea or water if you feel hungry later in the evening. If you must snack, have a vegetable with a low GI.

Throughout the day, drink plenty of water. Make sure to make and stick to a regular sleep schedule.

If you will be out of the house, at work or doing errands, make sure to bring a portable, healthy snack with you. Good choices include celery sticks or baby carrots with peanut butter, or apples.

On the days that you don't do an aerobic workout, make sure to get some form of exercise. For example, you might do some yoga or Pilates, or just take a long walk with your dog.

Week Two

Pay careful attention to the percentage of micronutrients you eat. Until you get used to this new way of eating, you may need to get a small kitchen scale and weigh your food. Remember that you should limit your intake of carb-rich foods like grains and starches to less than 25% -- and if you have a lot of weight to lose you should keep that number under 15%. Eat carb-rich foods early in the day and after you work out.

Your optimal day would include:

1 serving of carb-rich food at breakfast, along with a healthy combination of low GI fruits and vegetables and lean protein.
A small snack before working out – an apple is a good choice.
A carb-replenishing post-workout meal – on days when you do yoga or something that's not particularly strenuous, the need to replenish carbs will not be as high.

A mid-afternoon snack of something with a low GI, such as some raw veggies.
A healthy dinner with little or no carb-rich foods, eaten before 8:00

You should also make sure to sleep well and regularly, and to do what you can to minimize stress. Stress causes your body to produce the hormones adrenaline and cortisol, both of which cause your body to conserve energy – which also means they slow your metabolism.

As you can see, timing your carbohydrate intake can have a big impact on the way your body looks and feels. If you eat a big bowl of pasta or ice cream at night, your body is going to store those carbs as fat. However, if you eat them early in the day and after you work out, your body will use them as energy and to replenish your glycogen stores. That means that you'll lose weight more easily than you ever have before because you'll be giving your body the food it needs – when it needs it.

One final thing – remember that, when it comes to carb-rich foods, your body really only needs them after you have used a lot of energy and when you are preparing to use a lot of energy. That makes them the ideal food to prep for a fight or race, or to recover from a big expenditure of energy. They're not a good choice if you are going to be sitting around all day. Biologically, your body isn't equipped to deal with those carbs, and that's why they get stored as fat. Fortunately, by using the techniques in this book, you can overcome that tendency, burn the carbs you eat, and finally lose those extra pounds.

Chapter 8 – Low-Carb Recipes

A lot of people think of low-carb recipes as not being particularly good, but that's simply not true. The key to delicious low-carb meals is to choose quality ingredients that pack a nutritional punch, and then find ways to cook them to maximize their flavor.

You already know from the previous chapter that you can eat virtually unlimited amounts of vegetables with a low glycemic index. That means if you want to make a monster salad for lunch, you can – as long as you don't overdo it on calorie-laden toppings like salad dressing, cheese and bacon.

Here are a few quick and easy recipes that are very versatile and easy to make.

Healthy Breakfast Burrito

Ingredients:
Two eggs, or ½ cup of egg whites or egg substitute
¾ cup chopped veggies (your choice, but good options include mushrooms, broccoli, spinach, tomatoes, onions, and bell peppers)
1 whole-wheat or gluten-free tortilla
Salsa or hot sauce to taste
Non-stick cooking spray

Coat a frying pan with non-stick spray and let it heat. While it heats, crack and beat the eggs or measure the egg substitute. When the pan is hot, add the vegetables and let them cook until they are at your desired level of doneness. Pour the eggs over the vegetables and cook them, stirring to mix them with the vegetables. When the eggs are cooked through, which should take four or five minutes, spoon them into the tortilla and top them with salsa or hot sauce.

Note: you can switch this recipe up by changing the vegetables and seasonings you use. You can also eliminate the tortilla and cook these in muffin tins – just spray them and bake for about 20 minutes at 350.

Low GI Stir Fry

Ingredients:

1 c. broccoli, chopped into florets (frozen is fine)

1 c. mushrooms, sliced

1 c. sugar snap peas

½ onion, sliced thin

2 cloves garlic, sliced

½ lb. shrimp, cleaned and deveined

½ c. water chestnuts, drained

½ c. bean sprouts, drained

Non-fat cooking spray

Soy sauce, tamari sauce, or low-sugar stir-fry sauce to taste

½ c. brown rice, cooked

Spray a wok or cast iron skillet with cooking spray. Add the onion and garlic and cook until they start to soften. Add the broccoli and cook for 2-3 minutes on high heat, then add the mushrooms and sugar snap peas. Continue cooking until the vegetables are crisp tender. Remove them to a bowl, reapply cooking spray, and add the shrimp. Cook them until they are just pink, then add the vegetables together with the water chestnuts, bean sprouts, and sauce. Stir fry 2-3 minutes, or until everything is heated through. Serve over rice. Serves 2.

Like the burrito recipe, this one can be easily adapted. You could do a summer version with zucchini, tomatoes, carrots, and fresh herbs, for example, and substitute chicken or pork for the shrimp. You can also eliminate the rice if you choose.

Post-Workout Lunch

After a workout, it is important to replenish your body's stores of glycogen. One way to do that is to eat some carb-dense foods combined with protein and healthy fat. Here's a quick recipe you can have after a workout to replenish.

Ingredients:

1 c. quinoa

1 large tomato, chopped and seeded

½ c. cauliflower, chopped

½ red bell pepper, chopped

½ onion, diced

4 oz. chopped chicken or turkey breast

Chicken broth

Vinaigrette to taste

Cook the quinoa in chicken broth following the package directions. While it cooks, prep the vegetables and sauté them in a large pan with non-stick cooking spray. When the quinoa is cooked, it to the skillet along with the chopped chicken or turkey breast. Continue cooking until the ingredients are combined and the chicken is heated through. While it is still hot, add vinaigrette to taste. You can eat this dish

56 |

hot, or refrigerate it and have it available as a post-workout pick-me-up.

Quick and Easy Food Substitutions

One of the things that proves to be a challenge for people who are accustomed to eating a diet high in refined carbs is figuring out how to make healthy (and tasty) substitutions. Here are some hints:

- If you want to sweeten something, it is best to stay away from artificial sweeteners like saccharin, aspartame and acesulfame. Instead, use Stevia, which is all natural, or use a small amount of honey instead of table sugar.
- Cauliflower makes an excellent substitute for potatoes. It is delicious mashed, and you can also use it to

make things like pizza crust and even risotto – just pulse raw cauliflower in your food processor until the pieces are about the same size as rice.

■ Sweet potatoes have a fairly high glycemic index, but they're fine to eat in small amounts after a workout. They contain a lot of nutrients.

■ Many people are sensitive to the sugar (lactose) in milk. Almond milk and coconut milk make good, lactose-free substitutes. Just make sure to buy unsweetened varieties.

■ Don't overlook coconut oil and coconut flour as cooking substitutes. They both have health benefits and they are easy to find.

■ Lettuce wraps are a quick and guiltless substitute for tortillas, wraps, and breads. Almost anything you can put in a sandwich can be wrapped in a big lettuce leaf instead.

The main thing to remember is that you can find fun and creative ways to change up your favorite recipes. For example, I know someone who uses thin slices of eggplant and zucchini instead of lasagna noodles. That's a sensible substitute that allows you to enjoy a favorite dish without guilt.

<u>Conclusion</u>

Thank you for reading *Carbs: The No-Bullshit Guide to Ultimate Fat-Loss Transformation through the Use of Strategic Carbohydrate Timing and Techniques*. There are a lot of diet plans out there, and most of them won't do a thing to help you. This one will because it puts the focus where it should be – on giving your body the healthy fuel it needs to keep going.

Here's a quick recap of the key points of the book:

- Your body needs all three macronutrients – carbs, proteins, and fats – to be healthy.
- Carbohydrates are not the enemy. Most of your carb intake should come from fruits and vegetables with a low GI, while no more than 25% should come from carb-rich foods like starches and grains.
- Fats are not the enemy either. Minimize your intake of saturated fat, eliminates trans fat, and get no more than 30% of your calories from healthy

monounsaturated or polyunsaturated fat.

- The food you eat triggers hormonal responses in the body. By eating the right foods at the right times, you can keep your hormones balanced and your metabolism high.

- A healthy diet should include no more than 25% carb-rich foods, 25-30% low GI carbs, no more than 30% healthy fat, and between 20-40% protein depending on your activity level.

- Maintaining a healthy and positive mindset is just as important as eating the right foods.

- You need to move your body if you want to lose weight – ideally you should do 30 minutes of cardio three or four times a week, and strength and toning exercises in between.

- The best time to eat carb-rich foods is early in the day and after a workout.

Tips for Getting Started

Finally, here are a few quick tips for getting started:

1. Take a few days to get your mind in line with what you want to do. Do not think of this as a short-term change. Think of it as a new way of fueling your body, something you'll do for the rest of your life.
2. Get other people in your house on board. If you are going to be eliminating processed foods, you're going to have to negotiate the presence of those items in your home with other inhabitants. It's best to do this up front so you're not

confronted with unexpected Fritos in a weak moment.

3. Get rid of as many processed foods as you can. If others in your home insist on having them, try to segregate them from the food you eat so you're not tempted.
4. Stock up on healthy foods and snacks so you always have something that's good for you.
5. Set up a regular sleep and workout schedule and stick to it.
6. Don't forget to stay hydrated.

If you follow these steps, you will be on your way to a healthier, more attractive body in no time. Weight loss can feel impossible, especially if you've been following one fad plan after another. Now that you've opted in for my no-bullshit plan, you can be sure that you'll be successful.

If my book has added **value to you and you enjoyed it then please leave a review as it helps other customers decide if they wish to buy the book too. I thank you very much for purchasing and wish you the very best in your future! **

Printed in Great Britain
by Amazon